Exploring Lies Within Me

Delving into the Depths of secrets and Self-Deception

Mark lucas

Copyright

Table of contents

Introduction:Unveiling the Veil

There is a veil—a garment of deceit and delusion that hides the truth of who we are and what we believe—in the vastness of the human experience. Our journey's Introduction, appropriately named "Unveiling the Veil," is a call to action, a rallying cry for self-awareness and sincerity in a world awash in deceit.

Fundamentally, the Introduction establishes the groundwork for the path of transformation that is to come. It pushes readers to confront the unsettling facts that lie beneath the veneer of deceit that covers their view of reality. It's a path of self-awareness, development, and emancipation; it starts with having the guts to remove the masks that obstruct our view and accept the reality of who we are.

However, what is this veil we are referring to? It is the stories we tell ourselves, the masks we put on, and the illusions we cling to to protect ourselves from the uncomfortable truth. It is the narratives we tell ourselves about our identities and convictions, despite a wealth of contradictory information. The veil has the ability to influence our ideas, attitudes, and behaviors in ways we might not even be aware of, despite its sneaky nature.

Readers are encouraged to consider their encounters with deceit and illusion, to challenge the narratives they have been taught, and to accept the discomfort that comes with the truth throughout the Introduction. It's a trip of reflection and self-analysis when the masks of deceit are pulled aside and the unvarnished reality of who we are is revealed.

However, there are obstacles in the way of lifting the curtain. Faced with our inner shadows, it takes bravery to accept our shortcomings and inadequacies with grace and humility. It asks that we embrace the radical idea that we are enough, exactly as we are, and let go of the desire for approval from others.

Nevertheless, amid the uneasy self-examination, there is a deep sensation of release—a release from the bonds of self-criticism and self-doubt. Because we can only hope to unleash the transformational power of authenticity and walk in the light of our truth when we embrace the truth of who we are, imperfections and all.

Readers are left with a poignant reminder as the Introduction comes to an end: although the path of lifting the veil is not simple, it is worthwhile. We can only hope to realize the full potential of our actual selves and enter into our entirety by facing the veils that obstruct our vision.

Chapter 1: The Mask We Wear

In the grand theater of life, we all play the leading role, donning masks crafted from the fabric of societal expectations, personal insecurities, and the desire for acceptance. Chapter 1 delves deep into the intricacies of these masks, exploring their origins, their purpose, and the profound impact they have on our identities. At birth, we arrive as blank canvases, innocent and pure. Yet, as we navigate the labyrinth of existence, we quickly learn that the world demands conformity. From the moment we take our first breath, society begins to shape us, molding our thoughts, beliefs, and behaviors to fit neatly within its predefined boundaries. These societal norms become the foundation upon which we construct our masks, meticulously crafting each layer to conceal our vulnerabilities and insecurities. The mask serves as a shield, protecting us from the harsh realities of judgment and rejection. It allows us to navigate the complexities of human interaction with a sense of safety and control, presenting to the world a carefully curated version of ourselves deemed acceptable by societal standards. Behind this facade lies a labyrinth of complexity, where our true selves remain hidden, guarded by walls of fear and uncertainty. But what drives us to don these masks in the first place? The answer lies in our innate need for connection and belonging. From the moment we enter this world, we yearn to be seen, heard and understood. Yet, in a society that values conformity over individuality, we learn to sacrifice

authenticity in favor of acceptance. We trade our true
selves for the illusion of belonging, unaware of the toll it
takes on our psyche and spirit. As we grow older, the
lines between reality and illusion blur, and we become
entangled in a web of deceit of our own making. We lose
sight of who we truly are, drowning beneath the weight
of expectations and projections. The mask becomes our
identity, the lines between fiction and reality blurred
beyond recognition. But what happens when the mask
begins to crack, revealing glimpses of the truth hidden
beneath? It is in these moments of vulnerability that we
are confronted with the reality of our existence. We are
forced to confront the lies we have woven, the masks
we have worn, and the truths we have buried deep
within ourselves. Chapter 1 invites readers to peel back
the layers of their masks, to confront the illusions they
have created, and to embrace the truth that lies within. It
challenges us to question the narratives we have been
fed, to challenge the status quo, and to reclaim our
authenticity in a world that demands conformity. For
beneath the mask lies a treasure trove of untapped
potential, waiting to be unleashed. It is here, in the
depths of our true selves, that we find the courage to
stand tall, to speak our truth, and to live authentically. It
is here that we discover the power of vulnerability, the
beauty of imperfection, and the freedom that comes
from embracing our true selves. As Chapter 1 draws to
a close, readers are left with a powerful reminder: that
the journey to self-discovery is not always easy, but it is
always worth it. For in shedding the masks we wear, we

uncover the beauty of our humanity and the limitless
potential that lies within us all.

Chapter 2: Echoes of Deception

In the quiet corners of our minds, echoes of deception reverberate, shaping the very fabric of our reality. Chapter 2 delves into the labyrinth of lies we construct, exploring the insidious nature of self-deception and the profound impact it has on our lives. At its core, deception is a powerful tool—a double-edged sword that can be wielded with precision or wielded against us. It begins innocently enough, a whispered falsehood here, a half-truth there. Yet, with each utterance, the web of deceit grows denser, entangling us in a web of lies of our own making. But why do we deceive ourselves in the first place? The answer lies in our innate aversion to discomfort. We are creatures of habit, creatures of comfort, and when faced with the harsh realities of life, we seek refuge in the safety of deception. We convince ourselves that the lies we tell are harmless and that they serve a greater purpose, shielding us from pain and disappointment. Yet, as Chapter 2 reveals, the truth has a way of making itself known, no matter how deeply we bury it. Like a persistent echo, it whispers to us in the silence of the night, demanding to be heard. And as the echoes grow louder, we find ourselves confronted with the consequences of our deception—the fractured relationships, the shattered dreams, the hollow victories. But perhaps the most insidious form of deception is the lies we tell ourselves. We convince ourselves that we are unworthy of love, undeserving of success, that we are fundamentally flawed. These lies become our reality, shaping our thoughts, beliefs, and actions in ways we may not even realize. And yet, amidst the chaos of deception, there lies a glimmer of hope. For just as we have the power to deceive ourselves, so too do we have the power to uncover the truth. It begins with a willingness to confront our lies, to peel back the layers of deception, and to face the discomfort head-on. It is in these moments of truth that we find liberation and freedom from the shackles of self-deception. We are no longer bound by the lies we tell ourselves, no longer enslaved by the echoes of deception that haunt us. Instead, we embrace our truth, imperfect and flawed though it may be, and in doing so, we find a sense of peace and wholeness we never thought possible. Chapter 2 challenges readers to confront their echoes of deception, to question the narratives they have been fed, and to embrace the truth that lies within. It is a call to arms, a rallying cry for authenticity in a world drowning in deceit. As Chapter 2 draws to a close, readers are left with a powerful reminder: that the path to liberation begins with honesty, with a willingness to confront the lies we tell ourselves, and the courage to embrace our truth. Only then can we break free from the chains of deception and step into the light of our authenticity.

Chapter 3: The Anatomy of Self-Deception

In the intricate tapestry of the human psyche, lies a complex network of thoughts, beliefs, and emotions that often deceive us. Chapter 3 delves into the anatomy of self-deception, unraveling the intricate layers that cloak our true selves and exploring the mechanisms by which we deceive both ourselves and others. At its core, self-deception is a psychological defense mechanism—a way for our minds to protect us from the discomfort of reality. It manifests in myriad forms, from denial and rationalization to projection and distortion. Yet, regardless of its guise, the result is the same: a distorted perception of reality that shields us from the truth. But why do we deceive ourselves in the first place? The answer lies in our innate desire for self-preservation. When faced with unpleasant truths or uncomfortable emotions, our minds instinctively seek refuge in the safety of denial. We convince ourselves that what we perceive to be true is, in fact, false—that our actions are justified, our beliefs unassailable. Yet, as Chapter 3 reveals, the consequences of self-deception can be far-reaching. It erodes the very foundation of our relationships, breeding mistrust and resentment where there should be honesty and vulnerability. It distorts our perception of reality, leading us down a path of delusion and disillusionment. And perhaps most tragically, it robs us of the opportunity for growth and self-discovery. But what drives us to deceive ourselves in the first place? The answer, in part, lies in our inherent fear of the unknown. We cling to the familiar, even when it no longer serves us, because the alternative—stepping into the unknown—is far more terrifying. We would rather live in the comfort of our illusions than face the discomfort of truth. And yet, as Chapter 3 reminds us, the truth has a way of making itself known, no matter how deeply we bury it. It whispers to us in the stillness of the night, urging us to confront our self-deception and embrace the discomfort of reality. It is only through this process of self-examination that we can hope to break free from the chains of deception and step into the light of our authenticity. Chapter 3 challenges readers to confront their anatomy of self-deception, peel back the layers of illusion, and embrace the discomfort of truth. It is a call to arms, a rallying cry for honesty and self-awareness in a world drowning in deceit. As Chapter 3 draws to a close, readers are left with a powerful reminder: that the path to self-discovery begins with a willingness to confront our own self-deception and embrace the discomfort of truth. Only then can we hope to break free from the chains of illusion and step into the light of our authenticity.

Chapter 4: Layers of Illusion

Within the labyrinth of the human psyche lies an intricate tapestry of illusions, woven together by the threads of perception, belief, and experience. Chapter 4 peels back the layers of these illusions, revealing the complex interplay between reality and fantasy, and exploring the profound impact they have on our perception of the world and ourselves.

Illusion, by its very nature, is elusive—a mirage that dances on the edges of our consciousness, teasing us with promises of grandeur and escape. It is a seductive force, drawing us in with the allure of possibility, only to leave us grasping at shadows. Yet, despite its ephemeral nature, illusion holds a power over us—a power to shape our thoughts, beliefs, and actions in ways we may not even realize.

But what lies at the heart of these illusions? Chapter 4 posits that at their core, illusions are born from a fundamental misunderstanding of reality—a distortion of truth that serves to protect us from the discomfort of uncertainty. We convince ourselves that what we see is real, that what we believe is true, even when evidence to the contrary abounds.

Yet, as Chapter 4 reveals, the layers of illusion run deep, intertwining with every aspect of our lives. From the images we see in the media to the stories we tell ourselves about who we are, illusion shapes our perception of reality in ways both subtle and profound. It creates a world of smoke and mirrors, where truth is obscured by the haze of deception, and reality becomes a matter of interpretation.

But what happens when the illusions we cling to begin to crumble, revealing the stark reality beneath? It is in these moments of disillusionment that we are confronted with the true nature of our existence—the fragility of our beliefs, the impermanence of our illusions, and the raw beauty of reality laid bare.

And yet, amidst the rubble of shattered illusions, there lies an opportunity for growth and self-discovery. For it is when we strip away the layers of illusion that we can hope to uncover the truth that lies beneath—the truth of who we are, what we believe, and what truly matters.

Chapter 4 challenges readers to confront the layers of illusion that cloak their perception of reality, to question the narratives they have been fed, and to embrace the discomfort of truth. It is a call to arms, a rallying cry for authenticity and self-awareness in a world drowning in deception.

As Chapter 4 draws to a close, readers are left with a powerful reminder: that the path to self-discovery begins with a willingness to peel back the layers of illusion and embrace the discomfort of truth. Only then can we hope to break free from the chains of deception and step into the light of our authenticity?

Chapter 5: Unraveling the Truth

In the depths of our consciousness, lies a hidden treasure—the truth. Chapter 5 embarks on a journey of unraveling this truth, navigating through the labyrinth of deception and illusion to uncover the raw, unfiltered reality that lies beneath.

Truth is a multifaceted gem, shimmering with clarity and radiance yet shrouded in layers of obscurity. It is the bedrock upon which our lives are built, the compass that guides us through the turbulent waters of existence. And yet, despite its fundamental importance, truth is often elusive—a fleeting mirage that dances on the edges of our perception, teasing us with promises of understanding and enlightenment.

But what is truth, and how do we unravel its mysteries? Chapter 5 contends that truth is not a fixed point but rather a journey—a process of discovery that unfolds over time. It is a tapestry woven from the threads of experience, perception, and introspection, each thread contributing to the rich tapestry of our understanding.

Yet, as Chapter 5 reveals, the journey to uncovering the truth is not always easy. It requires courage, humility, and a willingness to confront our own biases and preconceptions. It demands that we peel back the layers of deception and illusion that cloak our perception of reality, exposing ourselves to the discomfort of uncertainty and vulnerability.

And yet, amidst the chaos of unraveling truth, there lies a profound sense of liberation—freedom from the shackles of deception and illusion that bind us, for it is when we embrace the discomfort of truth that we can hope to transcend the limitations of our understanding and step into the light of clarity and insight.

But the journey to unraveling truth does not end with mere discovery. It is a continuous process—a lifelong commitment to seeking understanding and enlightenment in the face of uncertainty and doubt. It requires us to remain open-minded and receptive to new ideas and perspectives, even when they challenge our deeply held beliefs.

As Chapter 5 draws to a close, readers are left with a powerful reminder: that the pursuit of truth is not a destination but rather a journey—a journey that requires courage, humility, and an unwavering commitment to authenticity and self-awareness. For only by unraveling the layers of deception and illusion that cloak our perception of reality can we hope to uncover the raw, unfiltered truth that lies beneath.

Chapter 6: Facing the Mirror

In the depths of self-reflection, lies the transformative power of Chapter 6: Facing the Mirror. This pivotal chapter delves into the profound act of introspection, exploring the journey of self-discovery and the transformative impact it has on our lives.

The mirror, both literal and metaphorical, serves as a portal to the soul—a reflection of our innermost thoughts, beliefs, and emotions. Yet, confronting the mirror can be a daunting task, as it forces us to confront the raw truth of who we are and who we aspire to be.

At its core, facing the mirror is an act of courage—a willingness to strip away the layers of deception and illusion that cloak our perception of reality. It is a journey into the depths of our psyche, where we confront our fears, insecurities, and vulnerabilities with unwavering honesty and authenticity.

But why is facing the mirror so important? Chapter 6 posits that self-reflection is the cornerstone of personal growth and self-awareness. It is through this process of introspection that we come to understand ourselves on a deeper level, unraveling the complexities of our psyche and uncovering the truth that lies beneath.

Yet, confronting the mirror is not without its challenges. It requires us to confront uncomfortable truths, to acknowledge our flaws and imperfections with humility and grace. It demands that we let go of the masks we wear, and the illusions we cling to, and embrace the raw, unfiltered truth of who we are.

And yet, amidst the discomfort of self-examination, there lies a profound sense of liberation—a freedom from the constraints of self-deception and illusion that bind us. It is when we face the mirror with courage and vulnerability that we can hope to transcend the limitations of our understanding and step into the light of authenticity and self-awareness.

But the journey of facing the mirror does not end with mere introspection. It is a continuous process—a lifelong commitment to self-discovery and personal growth. It requires us to cultivate a sense of curiosity and wonder about the complexities of our psyche, and to approach ourselves with compassion and empathy, even in the face of our shortcomings.

As Chapter 6 draws to a close, readers are left with a powerful reminder: that the journey of facing the mirror is not an easy one, but it is a journey worth taking. Only by confronting the raw truth of who we are can we hope to unlock the transformative power of self-discovery and step into the light of our authenticity.

Chapter 7: The Journey Inward

In the vast expanse of the universe, there exists a journey that transcends time and space—a journey of self-discovery that takes us to the very core of our being. Chapter 7: The Journey Inward embarks on this profound odyssey, exploring the depths of the human soul and the transformative power of introspection.

The journey inward begins with a single step—a moment of quiet reflection, where we turn our gaze away from the external world and direct it inward, towards the hidden recesses of our consciousness. It is a journey of self-exploration, where we confront the raw truth of who we are and who we aspire to be.

At its core, the journey inward is a quest for meaning and purpose—a search for understanding in a world filled with chaos and uncertainty. It is a journey of self-discovery, where we uncover the depths of our desires, fears, and aspirations, and come to a deeper understanding of the essence of our being.

But the journey inward is not without its challenges. It requires courage to confront the shadows that lurk within us and acknowledge our flaws and imperfections with humility and grace. It demands that we let go of the masks we wear, and the illusions we cling to, and embrace the raw, unfiltered truth of who we are.

And yet, amidst the darkness of self-examination, there lies a glimmer of hope—a beacon of light that guides us through the depths of our consciousness. It is only by confronting the shadows within us that we can hope to transcend them and emerge into the light of our authenticity and self-awareness.

But the journey inward is not just about confronting our demons—it is also about embracing the beauty and wonder of our existence. It is a journey of self-acceptance, where we come to appreciate the unique gifts and talents that make us who we are and recognize the inherent worth and dignity of every human being.

As Chapter 7 unfolds, readers are invited to embark on their journey inward—to explore the depths of their consciousness and uncover the hidden truths that lie within. It is a journey of self-discovery, personal growth, and transformation—a journey that holds the promise of a deeper understanding of ourselves and the world around us.

As Chapter 7 draws to a close, readers are left with a powerful reminder: that the journey inward is not just a destination, but a continuous process—a lifelong commitment to self-discovery and personal growth. For only by delving into the depths of our consciousness can we hope to unlock the true potential of our humanity and step into the light of our authenticity.

Chapter 8: Shadows of the Past

In the vast tapestry of our lives, the shadows of the past linger like ghosts, haunting our thoughts, shaping our beliefs, and influencing our actions. Chapter 8: Shadows of the Past delves into the profound impact of our personal histories, exploring how the echoes of yesterday continue to reverberate through the corridors of our minds.

The shadows of the past are not mere specters—they are the sum total of our experiences, both triumphs and tribulations, woven together into the fabric of our identity. They are the memories that linger, the wounds that never fully heal, and the lessons that shape who we are and who we aspire to be.

At its core, Chapter 8 delves into the complexities of memory and perception, exploring how the events of our past shape our understanding of ourselves and the world around us. It examines how we reinterpret our memories through the lens of our present experiences, constructing narratives that reflect our evolving sense of self.

But the shadows of the past are not always benevolent—they can also be the source of pain and trauma that linger long after the events that caused them have passed. They are the scars that mar our souls, the wounds that never fully heal, and the ghosts that haunt our dreams.

And yet, amidst the darkness of our past, there lies a glimmer of hope—a beacon of light that guides us through the shadows, for it is only by confronting the ghosts of our past that we can hope to transcend them and emerge into the light of our authenticity and self-awareness.

But the journey of confronting the shadows of the past is not an easy one. It requires courage to confront the wounds that lie buried beneath the surface and to acknowledge the pain and trauma that we have endured with humility and grace. It demands that we let go of the resentment and bitterness that bind us to the past and embrace the healing power of forgiveness and acceptance.

As Chapter 8 unfolds, readers are invited to confront the shadows of the past—to explore the depths of their personal histories and uncover the hidden truths that lie within. It is a journey of self-discovery, personal growth, and transformation—a journey that holds the promise of healing and liberation.

As Chapter 8 draws to a close, readers are left with a powerful reminder: that the shadows of the past do not define us—they are but a part of the rich tapestry of our lives. For only by confronting the ghosts of our past can we hope to break free from their grip and step into the light of our authenticity and self-awareness.

Chapter 9: Embracing Authenticity

In a world inundated with facades and illusions, Chapter 9 invites us to shed the masks we wear and embrace the liberating power of authenticity. It delves into the profound journey of self-discovery, urging us to peel back the layers of deception and embrace the truth of who we are at our core.

Authenticity is not a destination but a way of being—a state of alignment between our inner truths and outer expressions. It is the courage to show up as our true selves, unapologetically and unabashedly, regardless of the expectations or judgments of others. And yet, despite its inherent simplicity, authenticity remains a rare and precious commodity in today's world.

At its core, Chapter 9 challenges us to confront the barriers that stand in the way of authenticity—the fears, insecurities, and societal pressures that compel us to hide behind masks of conformity. It examines how we betray ourselves in pursuit of acceptance, sacrificing our truth on the altar of social approval.

But the journey of embracing authenticity is not without its challenges. It requires courage to confront the shadows that lurk within us and to acknowledge the vulnerabilities and imperfections that make us human. It demands that we let go of the need for external validation and embrace the radical notion that we are worthy of love and belonging simply by our existence.

And yet, amidst the uncertainty of self-discovery, there lies a profound sense of liberation—a freedom from the constraints of self-doubt and self-criticism that bind us. It is when we embrace the truth of who we are, flaws and all, that we can hope to unlock the transformative power of authenticity and step into the light of our truth.

But the journey of embracing authenticity does not end with mere self-acceptance. It is a continuous process—a lifelong commitment to self-discovery and personal growth. It requires us to cultivate a sense of curiosity and wonder about the complexities of our psyche, and to approach ourselves and others with compassion and empathy.

As Chapter 9 unfolds, readers are invited to embark on their journey of embracing authenticity—to explore the depths of their consciousness and uncover the hidden truths that lie within. It is a journey of self-discovery, personal growth, and transformation—a journey that holds the promise of liberation and wholeness.

As Chapter 9 draws to a close, readers are left with a powerful reminder: that authenticity is not a destination but a way of being—a choice we make every day to show up as our true selves in a world that often demands conformity. Only by embracing the truth of who

we are can we hope to unlock the transformative power
of authenticity and step into the light of our truth.

Chapter 10: Liberation of the Self

In the culmination of our journey, Chapter 10 beckons us towards the ultimate liberation—the liberation of the self. It is a chapter that embodies the essence of freedom, urging us to break free from the chains of self-imposed limitations and societal expectations and to embrace the boundless potential of our authentic selves.

At its core, the liberation of the self is a journey of empowerment—a reclaiming of our inherent worth and dignity as human beings. It is the recognition that we are not defined by our past or our circumstances but by the choices we make and the values we uphold. It is the realization that true freedom lies not in conforming to the expectations of others, but in embracing the truth of who we are and living in alignment with our deepest values and aspirations.

But the path to self-liberation is not always easy. It requires courage to confront the fears and insecurities that hold us back, to challenge the limiting beliefs that have been instilled in us since childhood, and to step boldly into the unknown. It demands that we let go of the need for external validation and embrace the radical notion that we are worthy of love and acceptance simply by our existence.

And yet, amidst the uncertainty and discomfort of
self-liberation, there lies a profound sense of
empowerment—a recognition of our own agency and
autonomy in shaping the course of our lives. It is only
when we free ourselves from the constraints of
self-doubt and self-criticism that we can hope to unlock
the true potential of our authentic selves and step into
the fullness of our being.

But the liberation of the self is not just about personal
empowerment—it is also about collective liberation. It is
the recognition that we are all interconnected, and that
true freedom cannot be achieved until all beings are
free. It is the commitment to social justice and equality,
and the willingness to stand up and speak out against
injustice wherever it may be found.

As Chapter 10 unfolds, readers are invited to embark on
their journey of self-liberation—to break free from the
constraints of self-doubt and self-criticism, and to
embrace the truth of who they are with courage and
conviction. It is a journey of self-discovery, personal
growth, and transformation—a journey that holds the
promise of a more liberated and empowered way of
being in the world.

As Chapter 10 draws to a close, readers are left with a
powerful reminder: that true freedom lies not in
conforming to the expectations of others, but in
embracing the truth of who we are and living in
alignment with our deepest values and aspirations. For

only by liberating ourselves from the constraints of self-imposed limitations can we hope to unlock the boundless potential of our authentic selves and step into the fullness of our being.

Conclusion: The Truth That Sets Us Free

In the grand tapestry of life, amidst the complexities of existence, one undeniable truth emerges—the truth that sets us free. Throughout our journey together, we have explored the depths of our consciousness, confronted the shadows of our past, and embraced the liberating power of authenticity. And now, as we stand at the threshold of our truth, we are reminded of the profound liberation that comes from embracing the truth of who we are.

The truth, elusive yet undeniable, is the cornerstone of our existence. It is the bedrock upon which our lives are built, the compass that guides us through the turbulent waters of existence. And yet, despite its fundamental importance, the truth is often obscured by layers of deception, illusion, and self-doubt. It is only by peeling back these layers, by confronting the shadows that lurk within us, that we can hope to uncover the truth that sets us free.

But what is this truth that we seek? It is the truth of our authenticity—the recognition that we are worthy of love and acceptance simply by virtue of our existence. It is the truth of our interconnectedness—the realization that we are all part of a larger whole, bound together by the common thread of humanity. It is the truth of our inherent worth and dignity—the understanding that we are not defined by our past or our circumstances, but by the choices we make and the values we uphold.

The truth that sets us free is not always easy to confront. It requires courage to confront the shadows of our past, to challenge the limiting beliefs that hold us back, and to step boldly into the unknown. It demands that we let go of the need for external validation and embrace the radical notion that we are enough, just as we are. But the rewards of embracing this truth are immeasurable—for in doing so, we unlock the boundless potential of our authentic selves and step into the fullness of our being.

As we journey forward, let us carry with us the wisdom gained from our exploration of truth. Let us remember that the path to liberation is not a solitary one, but a collective journey that we embark on together. Let us stand in solidarity with one another, supporting and uplifting each other as we navigate the complexities of existence.

And let us never forget the transformative power of truth—the truth that sets us free. It is only by embracing the truth of who we are, with courage and conviction, that we can hope to unlock the true potential of our authentic selves and step into the fullness of our being.

www.ingramcontent.com/pod-product-compliance
Lightning Source LLC
Chambersburg PA
CBHW071004250726
48663CB00002B/368